The ABZZZ's of Sleep: Insomnia, Sleep Apnea & Other Sleeping Disorders

A Definitive Guide for Problematic Sleepers

By: Dr. James Kohan

Speedy Publishing LLC

2658 Del Mar Hts Rd, #358
Del Mar, CA 92014
www.SleepDisordersInformation.org

DISCLAIMER

This book is not intended as medical advice. It is also not intended to
prevent, diagnose, treat or cure disease. Instead the book is intended only
to share the unofficial research and opinion of the author. The information
is provided for educational purposes only, not as treatment instructions for
any disease or ailment. Much of the book is a statement of opinion in areas
where the facts are controversial or do not exist. The information in this
book should not be considered any more valid than any other type of
informal opinion.

The information was not written to replace the advice or care of a qualified
health care professional. Be sure to check with your own qualified health
care provider before beginning any protocols or procedures discussed in
this book, or before stopping or altering any diet, lifestyle, or other
therapies previously recommended to you by your health care provider.

The treatments described in this book may have side effects and carry
other known and unknown risks and health hazards.The statements in this
book have not been evaluated by the United States FDA. Use of the
information in this book is at your own risk.

This book is dedicated to all the sleepless who suffer in silence.

"Sleep is the best meditation."
—Dalai Lama

A MESSAGE TO ALL SLEEPLESS SOULS

Sleeping is one of life's simplest and most relaxing pleasures. I say pleasure because, in all honesty, that's what it truly is. When we sleep, our body benefits from it the most. I am Dr. James Kohan and for the better part of three decades, I have been studying sleep and all its aspects —more so to help those who are in dire need of it. In years of study and working with patients I've found two critical benefits to sleep:

Dreaming. When your body enters a relaxed state and you slowly drift into unconsciousness, you get to experience what is usually known as R.E.M. This phase in sleep allows you to dream. While dreaming might seem mundane, in reality, it's what keeps you thinking, learning and remembering more fully. It allows you to experience life more fully through your sense and emotion, as well as to concentrate and direct your attention. Without dreaming, the brain would never be able to deal with all the stimulation that it receives each and every second of the waking day.

Rejuvenation. Sleep offers our bodies sanctuary from all the waking activities we perform. Like it or not, the body is like a machine —subject to wear and tear— and if not taken cared of properly, would deteriorate and diminish in performance before its supposed time. A good amount of quality sleep keeps you going every single day.

If you find yourself with difficulties in falling asleep or staying asleep, or are cranky, moody, slow on the uptake and generally lack an ability to go about daily activities, then relax —you are in the right place. After thousands of patients, I understand —you are NOT to blame! You are simply exhausted —physically & mentally.

I've dedicated my life's learning and medical practice to helping people with sleep problems. If you are anxious for answers right away, download *Sleep Soundly: Fall Asleep In Five Easy Steps* as my gift to you (retails for $9.99):

http://SleepDisordersInformation.org/sign-up

Here's a chance to reclaim what is rightfully yours… your rest, rejuvenation and relaxation! Loss of sleep and/or the inability to have any (consistent quality sleep) can be more detrimental to your health than you might be willing to recognize. I earnestly hope that by reading this book, you will find yourself in the arms of restful slumber once more. For all your inquiries on how to sleep soundly, I'm here to help. Feel free to send me an email.

All the best,
Dr. James Kohan
dr.jameskohan@sleepdisordersinformation.org

TABLE OF CONTENTS

INTRODUCTION

We spend 1/3 of our lives sleeping! The math adds up, but can you believe that something which should be so much a part of our lives is given so little "time." For comparison, we should spend 1/8 of our lives eating, but that seems to be getting a lot more attention. How many food channels, talk showsand everyday conversations that are centered around what we eat, what we're eatingand what we will eat, do we have? Not to mention, the topics of eating too much, too little or the right and wrong amounts, most of which comes back to health. The world of health information is exploding before our eyes and ears.

This brings us to sleep —not only is it our escape from the pressures of living, our quiet companion from its joys andtribulations, but the harbinger of good health and healthy living itself. For what doesn't go better with a good night's sleep? The gratitude of life's pleasures is better appreciated, the challenges of life's setbacks better tolerated and experienced.For what is sleep, if not simply, a time and period for our bodies to replenish themselves, a chance to dream and hopefully be more apt to start living life the next day.

Over 500 years ago, Sir Francis Bacon said, "Silence is the sleep that nourishes our wisdom." However, sleep is also the silent time of our lives. Even someone with a life threatening sleep disorder will not know it. How could they, as they are "sleeping?" We think that we would be awakened if something was wrong, but that is not usually the case, or it may happen too late.Even with a good medical checkup, including daytime tests, the body's systems may not work properly during sleep. When the body goes to sleep, all of its systems including the heart, lungs, brain, nerves and circulation do not "go to sleep." They have to keep working down to the cellular level and, sometimes, the challenges are more stressful during sleep compared to anytime during the day.

So sleep is not just a luxury item in life, it isn't something that can be sacrificed at any time to "add to the waking hours." For while sleep can be viewed as a refuge or even a reward for a good day's work, sleep will always be a necessity of life, moreso than any meal, with nearly as much significance as any breath of air or heartbeat.

CHAPTER 1- DEFINING SLEEP PATTERNS

How can you tell if someone is sleeping or not? They may look as if they are in a deep sleep but there is more to it than just looking. Everyone has brain waves and you can't tell when someone is in deep sleep by just looking at them. Through these brain waves, the different stages of sleep can be determined.

Expect Changes

Following being fully awake there is a transition stage. Then there are three stage of sleep; we call them: light sleep, deep sleep and dream sleep. Dream sleep is very different from the other stages of sleep. It is also very different from wakefulness, such that, we consider there to be three separate states of consciousness: awake, non-dream sleep and dream sleep.

When a person goes to sleep, the brainwaves slow down and enter the first stage of sleep known as the alpha rhythm which is a brief transition into a light sleep. When this happens, the brainwaves experience little voltage "kicks", or "K complexes, and it is an indication that the person is in a light sleep. Now we can say, "The person is asleep".

Throughout the night, a sleep evolves as the voltage increases and the speed of the brain waves slows down. This is the progression into "deep" sleep. This indicates that the person is very relaxed and in a deep sleep and it will not be easy to wake them up.

In "deep" sleep the body becomes limp, the muscles are relaxed and the breathing, heart rate and metabolism become slower. This is our more relaxed and restful stage of sleep. The next stage is "dream" or REM sleep wherein the brain waves speed up again but the body becomes paralyzed. At this point, a person stops moving, losing control of their temperature which renders us to be like a cold-blooded animal.

In addition, during "light" and "deep" sleep, the brain monitors the person's carbon dioxide and oxygen level so it can speed up or slow down the breathing and keep both the carbon dioxide and oxygen at set levels. However, in "dream" sleep, the brain will allow both O_2 and CO_2 to drift beyond "safe" awake levels. This condition is not entirely safe but it is what happens when a person dreams because the brain has a primitive desire to "dream" and thereby ceases to closely monitor parts of the body. Only when more extreme levels of temperature and O_2/CO_2 levels are reached will the brain "alert" itself.

When people are dreaming, the only muscles that continue to work are the eye muscles and the breathing diaphragm muscle. The eyes develop a rapid eye movement (REM) and move back & forth in a scanning motion. This is normal in dream sleep and is why it is called the "REM" sleep. The breathing diaphragm continues to work alone during "REM" sleep; when awake or in the other non-REM stages, the diaphragm is assisted by other chest, back, neck, and throat muscle during the breathing process.

As a sleep develops through the night, the light sleep will then progress to deep sleep in "cycles". Sleep progresses from awake to light sleep, to deep sleep to dream sleep, and then back to awake, every 60-90 minutes. Therefore, it is quite normal to wake up five or six times a night (or every 60 to 90 minutes). Fortunately, we usually fall back into sleep within a few minutes so we don't remember these awakenings. Studies have shown that you have to be awake for 8 to 12 minutes in order to remember it! There are also different patterns to this sleep cycle as the night progresses. "Deep" sleep is usually experienced during the first half of the night and the first cycle from awake to dream sleep is when people get most of their deep sleep. "REM" sleep occurs more in the second half of the night, and our longest REM sleep occurs just before we wake up. This last "dream" session can last up to 20 minutes! So in general, there are less "deep" sleep episodes and more "dream" sleep as the night passes. However, this pattern does change as we age.

In the first cycle, people may dream for a minute or two. But as the clock ticks on and gets nearer to the time a person needs to wake up, a dream may occur for twenty minutes which is a long time for the brain to not monitor the body. Although this happens, there is nothing to worry about because these changes in sleep patterns take place every night in the course of a lifetime.

ABZZZ's of Sleep

A newborn baby often sleeps for 16 hours or more in a day and dreams 50% of the time it is asleep. The up until the late teens or early twenties, the amount of dream sleep decreases and only takes up 20% of the total sleep time. This 20% REM pattern will then continue for the rest of our life. Young children who are still growing get a lot of deep sleep and that does not start going down until they reach the age of twenty-five. At that age, the amount of deep sleep starts to reduce so that by the age of 40, the amount of deep sleep drops by half.

Sixty-year-olds and above only experience a deep sleep for about 5% of the time they are asleep but their light sleep pattern increases and their dream sleep remains about the same. During "Deep" sleep growth hormone is secreted by the brain, so young children are the ones who need& get the most deep sleep. They also progress very quickly from awake to deep sleep, almost bypassing the normal progression through light sleep. This is why we see very active young children fall asleep so quickly when they "slow" down in a relaxed quiet atmosphere, like in a car seat! Their rapid progression into "deep" sleep is why they become so limp and are difficult to wake up (fortunately; right, mom & dad!). This is quite natural as they experience "deep" sleep when the brain waves are slow and the body most relaxed.

When people start complaining that they don't sleep as well as they used to, it just means their sleep pattern has changed. In fact, they are right! Although they are sleeping for the same amount of time, they are not getting as much "deep" sleep as they used to and in its place they get more "light" sleep. Unfortunately, this means that it is easier to be awakened, corresponding to the names "light" and "deep" sleep.

A truck or a car outside their house or any sudden noise might wake people up when they are older while a child would probably sleep through it. This is one of the reasons older people do not sleep as well as they used to when they were younger.

So it may be said that the key to a better night's sleep relates to getting more "deep" sleep. The best way to get more "deep" sleep is be more active during wakefulness. Studies have shown that people who do manual labor or exercise more vigorously get more "deep" sleep. So some simple advise for getting better sleep is to be more active, give up some conveniences of everyday life (car, elevator, leaf blower), and exercise regularly.

Chapter 2- The Consequences of Sleep Disorders

There are plenty of things that can go wrong with our sleep, many of whichcan affect our wakefulness as well. In order to understand sleep disorders, a simple separation into four general categories will be helpful.

Four Things That Can Go Wrong With Sleep
• Having trouble going to sleep and not getting enough sleep
• Excessive daytime sleepiness or somnolence
• "Parasomnia"- an unwanted behavior which occurs during sleep
• Sleep-wake disorders or circadian rhythm disorders

Insomnia

Is a symptom or group of symptoms which causes people to have problems going to sleep, staying asleep, or awakens them from it too early. When people suffer from insomnia they feel very tired the following day and they cannot function well. They have trouble thinking straight and cannot get any job done properly.They feel irritable and sometimes have difficulty adapting to stressful situations. Interpersonal relations can be strained. In short, insomnia affects every aspect of the waking day. Trouble falling asleep is called "sleep-onset Insomnia." Difficulty staying asleep is called "sleep maintenance Insomnia." Waking up too early is called "early awakening Insomnia." While many people with insomnia have aspects of each type, categorizing insomnia in this manner can frequently help with determining the most likely cause and,more often than not, help with a treatment solution. While insomnia sufferers can feel tired during the daytime, they are usually bothered more by the feeling of irritability or anxiety. Insomnia is the most common complaint related to sleep, estimating as many as 40% of the population, complaining about having trouble falling or staying asleep on any given day. 10% of the total population suffers from chronic insomnia. Most people suffering from insomnia tend to "suffer in silence,"thereby limitingtheir treatment to self-medication with "over-the-counter" or home remedies.

Excessive daytime somnolence

This is a common problem affecting people.Those with this problem usually feel like they are "fighting off sleep" all day long. They have difficulty with concentration and memory. While many of the people with this type of sleep problem feel like they slept all night and almost all will say that they have no problem *going to* sleep. The real cause of excessive daytime sleepiness *is* the **quality** of sleep overnight. The amount of sleep is usually not the main problem with *excessive daytime somnolence.* People who suffer from this affliction usually have no trouble falling asleep. In fact, with any reduction in daytime stimulation, the sufferer of excessive daytime somnolence will usually doze off.

One of the main causes of this is called sleep apnea. While this condition has been known for many centuries, it has only been commonly diagnosed and its treatment advanced over the past 40 years. Now, sleep apnea is the most common disorder seen and treated by sleep specialists.

Those suffering from sleep apnea stop breathing while they are asleep. There are two types of *sleep apnea. Centralsleep apnea* results when the brain stops sending the signal to breath to the respiratory muscles. In *Obstructive sleep apnea*, the signal to breath continues but the muscles of the throat and airway above the voice box (Larynx) relaxes too much and "obstructs" the flow of air into the lungs. Obstructivesleep apnea is by far the more common type of sleep apnea.

During the 1970s, doctors who worked in the pulmonary or respiratory section of medicine began to study breathing patterns of people while they slept and became very interested in what happens to people suffering from a lung condition when they fall asleep. As mentioned earlier, people who go into a deep sleep find their muscles totally relaxed while those in dream sleep become paralyzed and cannot move. So people with *"daytime"* lung conditions were seen to have low oxygen levels whenever they were in "deep" or "REM" sleep, corresponding to a time when their respiratory muscles were either very relaxed("deep" sleep) or paralyzed("REM" sleep). From this interest in breathing and sleep, the discovery of sleep apnea as a separate disease was made and advanced. You see, sleep apnea *is not* a lung disease, per se. It *is* a breathing disorder. The lungs are normal in people with only sleep apnea.

In the last 40 years, this is how sleep medicine became a major part of pulmonary medicine. Like me, most of today's sleep specialists started their medical careers as pulmonary doctors. It was the discovery of sleep apnea and the surprising frequency of its occurrence that has spurred the growth of sleep medicine over the past 3decades. Thirty years ago, people had heard of sleep apnea but did not know anyone who suffered from the problem. It has become more common in the last 20 years and today all doctors and medical students are trained on how to diagnose and treat sleep apnea. Of course, many of this would not be possible if not for the many technological advances that have allowed us to study people while they sleep *without* their sleep being affected much by the process used to study it. In short, the instruments used to study sleep have become smaller, lighter, and more accurate.

Sleep apnea is now a very common condition and cannot be ignored as it affects the sufferer's general health. Even if people are extremely healthy during the day, if they have severe sleep problems during the night, they should still be assessed for sleep apnea. If there are any breathing problems (or heart or circulation problems) during the day, they will get worse at night with sleep. Thus, medical attention is necessary. Many times, cardiac, psychiatric, Infectious or endocrine diseases can be optimally treated, yet nocturnal/ sleep related worsening can still be occurring with gradual yet unforeseen deterioration which is unavoidable if underlying sleep apnea is not diagnosed and treated.

People suffering from sleep apnea can stop breathing for at least 10 seconds and as long as 90 seconds at a time. They do this repeatedly throughout the night, and can happen every night or whenever they sleep.

The most common way to determine if someone has sleep apnea is whether they are extremely tired in the daytime. Another way of telling if someone suffers from the problem is when they snore loudly at night. The combination of daytime sleepiness and nighttime snoring is a telltale sign.

Snoring is caused by the muscles of the throat becoming obstructed. Obstructive sleep apnea or OSA, as it is known, happens when people go into a deep sleep and the throat muscles relax or when they go into dream sleep and the throat muscles become paralyzed. (The "upper" airway, that part above the windpipe (trachea), is a muscular channel from the back of the nose down to the top of the voice box (larynx). When this takes place, the throat collapses and the diameter of the throat opening is reduced by 50% or more for 10 seconds. The throat closes down, the flow stops and the snoring becomes louder because of the "flapping" of the walls at the back of the throat. The tongue relaxes and the throat muscles alternate between vibration and relaxation. The smaller the throat opening is, the louder the snore. Because of this collapse, the amount of air in the lungs is reduced, and the oxygen in the blood begins to fall for anything between a few seconds to a full minute. As the oxygen falls, the brain realizes the oxygen is dropping, and sends a signal down to the "upper" airway/throat muscles to awaken. This happens because the brain bumps itself into a lighter stage of sleep; either "Light" sleep or briefly awake. These muscles awaken, but the sleeper doesn't. The sleeper usually briefly "grunts" or "snorts" and the flow of air is restored to the lungs.

This type of wakefulness means the person is not fully awake but the sleep pattern is lightened. The brain is responsible for stopping the apnea because it has noticed the falling oxygen levels and has bumped the person back into a light sleep or semi-wakefulness. The main problem for sleep apnea sufferers is every time this happens, the body is put under stress as the oxygen falls before the brain kicks in and the heart is robbed of oxygen. The lungs realize there is less oxygen than usual in them and the blood pressure rises in the lungs. The heart rate gets slower to save oxygen before panicking and speeding up again, thus, sending the blood pressure in the arms and legs shooting up. This sudden shift from a slowing of the heart into a panicked state with elevated BP and racing heart rate can lead to life threatening heart rhythm disturbances and sudden death. "He died in his sleep" can frequently mean undiagnosed and untreated Sleep Apnea.

This is the "physiologic" danger of sleep apnea: high blood pressure, heart attack, and stroke. They also have the problem of not getting enough deep sleep due to the brain continuously bumping them back into a light sleep. Every time the brain wants to return to a deep sleep, the throat collapses and the snoring gets louder and so the cycle continues. As the best sleep you can get is deep sleep, the older sufferers find that the deep sleep they achieve that is already reduced by age is reduced even further. The person with Sleep Apnea rarely if ever gets any "deep" sleep, so they never feel rested the next day, *no matter how long they sleep.* Apneas or stopping breathing can occur anywhere from a minimum of 5 to10 times an hour up to worst cases of 80 times an hour.

Normally people only wake up from sleep every 90 minutes but sleep apnea sufferers cannot remain in a deep sleep because they are being bumped into wakefulness every 1to 6 minutes all through the night.

They are unaware of this constant disruption because they remain in some form of sleep, albeit a "light" sleep at best.

Another way of trying to understand how this feels is to imagine that while you are sleeping somebody is shaking you all through the night. You are shaken on the shoulder and you shrug it off but the following day you remember nothing about it and just feel that you "have not slept all night". In most cases, sleep apnea may not be life-threatening but it is very inconvenient and disruptive to the smooth sleep transitions that should usually make people feel great when they wake up.

Parasomnia

"Things that go bump in the night". Examples are sleepwalking, sleep talking, night terrors and bed wetting. These can be considered "normal" and part of the development in children or they can also occur in adults. Further insight and understanding will be discussed in a later chapter.

Sleep-Wake schedule or Circadian rhythm disorders

Are common in the general population and most of which are usually self adjusting or well tolerated for brief periods. Examples are "jet lag" and "shift work" problems. However, with more extensive air travel and the frequency of shift work throughout the world, these problems are becoming more pervasive. These will be discussed in a later chapter.

Chapter 3- Children's Sleep Patterns

Sleep patterns change throughout our lifetime, but mostly during the first twenty years. Differences in sleep occur especially during our early childhood. While it's not surprising to learn that newborn infants sleep for up to 16 hours per day, did you know that babies spend 50% of their sleeping time in dream (REM) sleep? During REM sleep, the babies' brain and nervous system is developing and in the first year of life, the most demanding changes occur. Think of how little a baby can do at birth —coo, breath, suck for food, poop— and then, by age 1 year old how much has changed. This is all related to the brain and nervous system's maturation. This is why the brain devotes so much energy to dream sleep in the first year of life. After the first year, the percentage of dream sleep is reduced and the amount of "deep" sleep increases. During deep sleep there is time for muscular growth and regeneration. This is also the time when the growth hormone is secreted by the brain. The growth hormone is the chemical that causes our muscles to grow in reaction to exercise and activity, and we all know how active children are. Think of how active a one year old is! This is the year when the body undergoes its most tremendous physical change and corresponds to a time when there's also the biggest change in the amount of "deep" sleep. After year one, the amount of sleep needed per 24 hours also starts to decrease in a yearly manner, such that a 1 year old needs 14-15 hrs of sleep per day. This is the amount over a 24 hr period, so that would include nap time as well as overnight sleep. Up until puberty, the amount of sleep per day reduces every year. This includes the percentage of "dream" sleep, with the increasing percentage of "deep" sleep making up the difference. So a 3 year old will need 12 to14 hours of sleep per day, a 7 year old will need 10-12 hours and a 12 year old will need 9 to 11 hours per day, and so on and so forth. This decreasing pattern of sleep requirement usually leads to a "nightly battle" over bedtime, up to, and, especially including the teenage years. "Well, I'm a year older now so I can stay up late for another hour," is the nightly cry of the school age child. And for the most part, they are right. A half hour less per year is probably more reasonable.

However, at puberty, the pattern not only stops but also reverses itself! A child going through puberty needs MORE sleep per day and sometimes up to 2 hours more than he or she did before puberty. This is because of the physical demands of the body undergoing so much change. Not since the first year of life has the body changed so much in such a short span of time. While there is a lot of "energy" associated with puberty, there is also much need for added sleep to allow recovery of the body each night (try telling this to a "child" who is used to going to bed at later times every night for the past 5 to 7 years)! Added to this is all the extra social activities (and "media") of the teenage years! Yet, during puberty and adolescence, the percentage of "deep" sleep will slightly increase and the percentage of "dream" sleep will slowly decrease to the adult level of 20% around the age of 20 years old. The percentage of "Dream" (REM) sleep will remain at 20% each night throughout the rest of life.

The different percentage and amount of each sleep stage accounts for many of the differences seen in the quality of sleep over time. In general, not only do children sleep more per 24 hours than adults do, but they spend more of their sleep in "deep" sleep. The percentage of "deep" sleep each night can be up to 30% during childhood, while adults have less percentage of "deep" sleep every year starting at about age 30 and declining throughout the rest of life (by age 60, less than 5% of our sleep is "deep" sleep)! Unfortunately for us adults, we do spend an INCREASING percent of our sleep in "light" sleep during our adult years. This difference in "deep" vs. "light" sleep is the biggest reason why we sleep differently as we age. "I don't sleep as well as I used to," Is one of the earliest complaints of an "aging" adult. Now you know why! It's because you spend LESS time in "deep" sleep and MORE time in "light" sleep. Remember that "deep" sleep is the most relaxing stage of sleep and the stage that is most difficult to be awakened from. "Light" sleep is just that; easy to be awakened from, so it's a more "restless" sleep. So, an adult will be more prone to waking up due to "lighter" sound, light, noise, change in temperature, etc. Also, an ache or pain that a child sleeps through, will most likely awaken the adult (not to mention the fact that adults have more aches and pain... think arthritis, stomach ulcers, cough, chest pain, headaches, etc.). Then, there's "T.B." which is more common in adults, especially men. Not "tuberculosis", I'm talking about "tiny bladder".

You may hear some people say that they wish they could sleep like a baby. If they were able to choose which age group they could experience, a 10 to 12 year old age group would be the best, since this age group gets 30% of "deep" sleep, which is the most relaxing sleep anyone can experience. This is the age group with the most mature amount of activity and hence, the highest percent of "deep" sleep, during which the muscles are regenerating for the next day (unfortunately, this may be changing as our children are becoming more involved with passive video games and less likely to engage in spontaneous physical activity).

So, what can sleep do for you? As previously stated, there are three different stages: awake, non-dream sleep and dream sleep. When people are in dream sleep, the brain speeds up and the body becomes paralyzed. The brain "erases its tapes" and prepares for the next day's mental activity. It actually helps people think more clearly the following day. They'll also be in a much better mood with improved concentration and a clearer memory, making them more apt to learn and, more mentally, as well as emotionally alert, to face the new day. The "deep" sleep (or non-dream sleep) allows the muscles to not only rest but also regenerate in preparation for the next day. So, the more active you are on a given day, the more "deep" sleep you will tend to get on that night.

A person will not get enough deep sleep as they grow older unless they increase their exercise routine and use their bodies more. The body needs to be tired from leading an active life to get more deep sleep. When people lead a sedentary lifestyle as most workers do now, they will experience far less deep sleep than those who have a very active job. Regardless of the mental demand of their job, only physical work or exercise will result in more "deep" sleep. It has been shown in sleep lab studies that people who have heavy manual labor jobs and marathon runners who train every day, are able to have a higher percentage in the amount of "deep" sleep compared to those who lead sedentary lifestyles. Their deep sleep is much like those of pre-teen children. So, if you want to sleep "like you used to", you need to get more "deep" sleep, and the only way to do this is to be more active during the day. Likewise, the sedentary individual will frequently encounter a restless night, with the difficulty in "turning off" the mental activity they've been immersed in all day. More on this in the later chapters about insomnia...

CHAPTER 4- SLEEP APNEA AND HYPERTENSION

As mentioned, sleep apnea is a very common and disruptive sleep disorder that is diagnosed and treated in sleep laboratories. It causes behavioral problems as a result of excessive sleepiness such as an inability to cope, poor concentration and irritability. The more dangerous side effect of sleep apnea is hypertension. Approximately 80% of those suffering from sleep apnea have high blood pressure. Probably the greatest risk for sleep apnea is that the person suffering from it is usually unaware of it! They are usually the last one to know!

This hidden aspect of the disorder adds to the double damage of high blood pressure. With hypertension, usually, only a very high and sudden rise in blood pressure will cause symptoms, typically headaches and blurring visions. Therefore, the condition of hypertension develops over years and the "cause" of high blood pressure is usually unknown. This is what is called "essential" hypertension. Over the past 20 to 30 years, Obstructive Sleep Apnea (OSA) has been recognized as one of the more common "silent" causes of high blood pressure. One of the earlier studies found that people seen in a medical clinic with new onset hypertension and NO OTHER COMPLAINTS were offered a diagnostic sleep study. The people had NO trouble sleeping and didn't note any snoring issues. Yet, during their sleep studies, 20% of them had sleep apnea! The link between hypertension and cardio-vascular disease, as well as stroke, has been well known for decades. OSA has recently been calculated to be 3-4 times at greater risk for heart attack and stroke if left untreated. Even if someone's hypertension is "under good control", this may be only a daytime "reassurance", because with every episode of "apnea" during sleep, there is a corresponding necessary sudden rise in blood pressure. This happens because of the drop in blood levels of oxygen during apnea; the blood vessels "squeeze" tighter in response to this. With OSA, this process can happen anywhere from 5 to 75 times per hour during sleep.

Even when the daytime blood pressure is good and people are generally healthy, if they have sleep apnea they can also develop a common problem called Atrial fibrillation. Approximately 15-20% of people over the age of 65 suffer from this condition. In Atrial fibrillation, the heart beats in an IRREGULAR manner. Both the speed and rhythm is irregular. The heart skips beats and changes speeds. Sometimes, It can speed up very rapidly (usually with caffeine, cold tablets or dehydration) and lead to dizziness or collapse. If that rapid attack doesn't happen, it can be tolerated pretty well... even for years. However, if Atrial fibrillation occurs intermittently, it can result in blood clots forming silently in the heart. These clots can suddenly travel to the brain and cause a stroke. A stroke is a sudden loss of oxygen in one part of the brain; this will happen when a blood clot blocks an artery delivering blood (and oxygen) to the brain. That part of the brain will fail, usually resulting in paralysis of one side of the body, speech problems, or inability to swallow. Approximately 25% of those who develop "AFib" will suffer a stroke during their lifetime.

Now, Atrial Fibrillation is also a condition which can occur with NO OTHER APPARENT heart problems. This is referred to as "idiopathic" in the medical textbooks, which means, "cause unknown". Once again, Obstructive Sleep Apnea (OSA) has been shown to be an underlying cause of Atrial Fibrillation. So a person with OSA has two increased risks for suffering a stroke: Hypertension and Atrial Fibrillation.

They also have another risk

Those suffering from sleep apnea are also more likely to be overweight, which will get worse because people who cannot sleep tend to get up and raid the fridge to compensate. They will also choose sweets and carbohydrates for a short period as the high sugar content will make them feel better.

Tiredness in the daytime also tempt people to snack, eating cookies and sweets to make them feel more alert. There's a chemical reason for this —part of the brain contains leptin, which is the chemical that causes people to feel and think clearly. When they develop sleep apnea, the brain has difficulty making leptin, so when the chemical levels fall, people tend to overeat as it makes them feel better.

Once they start treatment for sleep apnea, they will start losing weight as the need to snack to be more alert will disappear. People with sleep apnea are also more likely to develop type 2 diabetes. This is the most common type and is due to people being overweight. One out of 10-20 people will suffer from sleep apnea, which broken down, is about 4% women and 10% adult men. And sleep apnea is as common as diabetes but not talked about as much.

Not only are diabetes and sleep apnea linked to being overweight, they are the most common medical problems around. It's like a vicious circle. When you have sleep apnea, you are more likely to put on weight, and the more weight you put on, the worse the sleep apnea gets, and this can continue throughout your lifetime. Men can develop sleep apnea in their early twenties and slowly they get more tired, so they overeat to compensate. In their thirties, they will put on a little more weight and the sleep apnea will go from being a very mild condition to a moderate or severe one between the ages of 25-50.

Women do not normally develop sleep apnea until their mid-late forties. However, the chances of getting sleep apnea increases especially after they menopause. The condition means you stop breathing for 10 seconds or more and the minimum time this happens is five every hour. If it is less than five, sufferers tend to think it is too mild to worry about. When doctors see a patient whose breathing stops between 5-15 times per hour, it is classified as mild sleep apnea. 15-20 times an hour is moderate and more than 25 times an hour is severe. As sufferers get older, their sleep apnea gets worse, and as it worsens with age and weight gain, so do their risk of having a stroke or heart attack.

CHAPTER 5- NIGHT AND SWING SHIFT WORK

"Shift work" is a modern phenomenon and has resulted in a separate sleep type of sleep problem. Due to the modernization of equipment ("machines don't get tired") and advances in lighting, 20% of the American work force operates overnight or as part of swing shifts. To briefly state the challenge, when you work at night, you are going against everything the brain considers to be normal. Yet, people who work these shifts frequently say they are "used to it" and think that little difference exists between night and day. When questioned further, they say, "I am a night person". Have they really adjusted their brains and body's natural way or are they missing something? When studies were carried out on night workers, it was discovered that their perceptions were wrong. People do not work as well at night, the job roles are actually reduced and the efficiency is not as good. More accidents at work happen during the night and industries have adopted strategies to take advantage of this. Psychologically, night workers are going against a natural behavior which makes the brain less alert and more likely to fall asleep, especially from 2AM to 5AM. It is during these times when people are most likely to fall asleep in a quiet room even if they have slept very well in the previous days. Anyone who has had to stay awake at night will say that is the time when they are least vigilant. However, part of the reduced vigilance (or alertness to changes around you) is the misperception that you are as alert as usual. In other words, the brain has a tendency to fool ourselves into thinking that we have "everything under control". Why is this so? Because you simply cannot sleep as well during the daytime as you would overnight.

If you compare someone sleeping for 7 hours during the day and someone sleeping for 7 hours during the night, you will find out that the person sleeping during the day gets 40% less sleep than the one sleeping during the night. They have less consistent sleep and less total amount of sleep during those 7 hours of "time in bed". They wake up more frequently and spend more time in a light sleep. Some of this is understandable as it is brighter and noisier in the daytime and there are more distractions. There is a lot of noise outside, noise from neighbors, more daytime transportation; let's face it, the rest of the world is awake and shows it by making all kinds of sound! Then, there are phone calls to also disrupt your sleep and it does not take much to disturb you because when you sleep, day or night, you have to cycle through not only "light" sleep, but also brief periods of awake. Night workers have been tested with portable sleep wave detection in their normal environment and this pattern of interrupted daytime sleep is observed over and over. There is also a pattern seen in inexperienced night workers where they tend to go to bed much later than veteran night workers. It is a natural tendency to feel more alert after the "normal" waking time, even if you've been up all night. Plus, there's a euphoric effect from having succeeded in "beating mother nature" by functioning all night long. This effect is the secretion of cortisol or adrenaline, which occurs normally each morning, and is part of the normal "circadian rhythm" of the brain & body. It is also triggered by the effects of morning sunlight.

To discuss further as to how the brain "fools us" into thinking that we are fully alert overnight, we must look more closely at how perception is affected by sleep stages. The first stage of sleep, or "light sleep", occurs readily in someone who is tired, even if they say that they are "awake". This can happen in short, brief episodes called "micro sleep", during which there may be only 20 to 60 seconds of "Light sleep" scattered between periods of being fully awake. The person would look no different during either degree of alertness, BUT they would be asleep during the brief "light" sleep moments. This means that they cannot see, hear, think or react normally. To add to the danger, they would not be able to "see" themselves as being asleep. Consider this! If you wake someone from a light sleep, 50% of them will deny that they were asleep and say they were just "resting". But if you asked them what has been happening while they were resting they will have no idea. Sleep lab experiments have been carried out where tired people have had their eyes taped open and they will go into a light sleep. They are then shown pictures on a screen or projector. When they are awakened, almost all of them will say they were not asleep. YET, they will not be able to recall seeing any of the pictures! This has been also done with sounds instead of pictures, and the results are the same. Proof that during "light" sleep, no matter how brief, the brain is not able to sense its surroundings and, it is the brain that fools them into thinking they are awake when the brain is actually sleeping. They are unable to take anything in or remember anything. This is the danger of light sleep, especially for someone who is operating equipment or driving a car wherein they could be in a light sleep and not know it and that is when accidents happen. Furthermore, there is the false sense of security that accompanies this misperception. Some people have experienced this when driving. They are tired and doze off without realizing it and when someone asks them if they had seen a road sign or an exit, they do not remember it. This is why most fatal car accidents happen between 2 and 6 AM, despite that being the time when there are the fewest cars on the road.

So the tired and less "vigilant" brain can go quickly In and out of light sleep and this is more likely to happen when we go against our natural day-night circadian rhythm. Night workers are going against the normal workings (physiology) of the brain. After the age of 40 this becomes more of a problem and it is not advisable for those over 40 to work night shifts. If you do have to work night shifts, certain tips can be helpful. First, don't think that you're "just staying up all night". You are not only working but you are challenging your brain and body in a very new and demanding way. Second, keep a regular sleep pattern and stick to it. Third, it is best to try and go to sleep as soon as possible after you get home. If possible, have someone else do the driving. Fourth, avoid exposure to early morning sunlight as this trigger the brain's "awake response". Wear sunglasses to leave work and get home, if at all possible. Fifth, avoid caffeine before sleep, but eat something to avoid hunger that might affect your daytime sleep. Sixth, provide a dark bedroom with no chance for sunlight to penetrate, even during later in the day. Seven, switch off timed appliances and silence (including vibrate) cell phones and voice mail receivers. Eight, sleep as long as you can. If you have to do things during the day, it is better to come home in AM, sleep for 4-5 hours, then get up and carry out your chores before returning to bed for 2-3 hours in evening before returning to work. This way you approach the total sleep time (up to 8 hours) that you would get when sleeping during the night. When you do have days off it is best to sleep a few hours in the AM but then go back to desired night sleep hours that first night. Regarding "swing shifts', it is best to rotate the shifts in a "forward fashion", such that you work a week's worth of "days", then a week of "evenings", then a week of "nights".

Remember, a tired brain and body is more prone to illness and accident, so if you have to work nights, be mindful of the challenges you are putting yourself through.

ABZZZ's of Sleep

CHAPTER 6- CIRCADIAN RHYTHM DISORDERS

The circadian rhythm is the cycle the brain adapts to both day and night. There is a gland the size of a pinhead that squirts out a chemical to help people adapt their life to sunlight and darkness. It is called the "pineal" gland, and the chemical is melatonin. This gland directs people to be more alert in sunshine and daylight and more relaxed or asleep when it gets dark. This is called the circadian rhythm and it works on a fixed pattern. If this pattern alters, it is usually caused by human behavior, not the brain. Common causes are jetlag (or travelling through different time zones rapidly) and working different shifts, especially night shifts or "swing" shifts. These cause our inner circadian rhythm to conflict with the light-dark cycle or "the clock on the wall". In these conditions, the brain continues to follow the "inner clock" which sets the circadian rhythm, while we are exposed or subjected to the "different" schedule around us.

There are two other conditions which involve circadian rhythm disturbances: the "delayed sleep phase syndrome" and the "advanced sleep phase syndrome". They normally affect two different groups of people. The delayed sleep phase happens to teenagers who stay up far too late at night and then cannot wake up in the morning while elderly people experience the advanced sleep phase which is caused by the opposite behavior. They go to bed too early and then wake up in the middle of the night.

The problem a teenager faces can be solved by altering their behavior pattern but this is not easy in a modern world as there are so many distractions to keep them awake late at night such as cell phones, computers and TV. When the teenager goes to bed in the early hours of the morning, sometimes as late as 4am, they are unable to wake up when everyone else wakes up and after a period of time their circadian rhythm changes. The brain gets confused by the teenager's sleep pattern and is unable to cope to this change in "sleep-wake" behavior. So the brain's behavior gets "delayed" in relation to the teen's behavior (and the clock on the wall), resulting in the teenager being awake when everyone is sleeping (late night/ early AM) and sleeping when everyone else is awake for the day (mornings). The teenager can't be awakened for school and will sleep on the bus and during morning classes. It is alarming and annoying for the parents who usually hope that by letting their teens sleep more on the weekend will solve the problem. But what happens is that the "delayed" circadian rhythm of the brain will just sleep later and then have to stay up even later that night before it is tired again. The problem is propagated; the cycle worsens. It's not unusual for teens with the delayed sleep phase syndrome to sleep until 2 pm or later.

To get back to the normal pattern, something has to be done to correct the problem but it is not easy. Worried mothers will take their "rebellious" teens to the sleep doctor, asking for advice and the problem can be solved in two ways. Call them the "1 day fix" or the "1 week fix". Both ways are hard for both parent and teenager, but this single attempt is more drastic as the teenager has to be kept awake for 36 hours, which means the parent has to stay awake as well. The child will not find a problem staying awake all night, but they have to remain awake throughout all of the following day and until the following night. NO NAPS are allowed (for teenage or their "monitor" parent.) In this manner the circadian rhythm will be "reset" back to normal. It is best to do this on a weekend when you can stay awake all Friday night and Saturday daytime and be very firm that they are not allowed to sleep during the day. The parent has to act like a warden and the teenager cannot be allowed to go to bed until the desired bedtime is reached. Usually 10 pm on the Saturday night when they can at last go to sleep. The teenager, who will be very tired by then will usually fall asleep easily and sleep through the entire night. When morning comes, the desired wake time should be sternly implemented.

The other alternative is to let the teenager stay up an hour longer every night until they reach the normal bedtime at around 10pm. For example, if the teenager has a habit of going to bed at 4 am, then the next night they are kept up until 5 AM, then allowed 8 hours sleep; the following night they are kept up until 6AM & allowed 8 hours sleep, etc. This is still difficult because they cannot be allowed to doze off at other times and it is a prolonged challenge for the whole family. This is best done during a school vacation or when there is 1 week of "free" time. Most families opt for the "1 day fix". The teenage years can be difficult for parents and children alike and it can have long-term consequences on the teenager if they are not fully alert during the day. The delayed sleep phase syndrome can result in a devastating semester for a student.

Fortunately, most teenagers only get delayed by 1-2 hours each day and by week's end they can "catch up" by sleeping an extra 2-4 hours on the weekend. Normally, the brain will sort itself out and adapt by the late teenage years but serious cases of circadian rhythm disorders need to be addressed.

The advanced sleep phase affects elderly people who go to bed too early in the evening (6-8PM) and wake up much too early in the AM (2-5AM), which is disruptive to other people living in the house. If they live alone or in a retirement home where they can set their own routine, this shouldn't matter. But if they are living with younger people or in a care home where they have a program of daytime activities, their brain needs to be on the same "sleep-wake" cycle as everyone else. The best way to cure this circadian rhythm disorder is to make sure the elderly person gets a lot of sunlight both in the morning and afternoon. This is not always possible in some parts of the country which do not get much sun but you can get lamps or "light boxes" which project artificial sunlight. 10,000 Lux brightness of white light or possibly 350-500 Lux of Blue or green light is needed. UV light needs to be filtered out to avoid eye damage. If the elderly person uses the lamp for 20 minutes in the late afternoon, it will help them stay awake longer, sleep through the night and the circadian rhythm will return toward normal. This could help avoid the high frequency of sleeping pills being used in adult care homes, which frequently results in elderly falls and hip fractures during the night and early AM hours.

CHAPTER 7- SLEEP PROBLEMS CAUSED BY JET LAG

As mentioned before, some sleep problems are caused by choice or habit. These include jetlag and working night shifts. As you travel across different time zones it is too fast for the brain to adapt so, when you cross two hour time zones the brain cannot take that in immediately. Travelling east is contrary to the tendency to just stay awake at night as you are effectively compressing the day. When you travel west, you are going to be more tired at night but you are going to wake up early in the morning; it is similar to the advanced sleep phase syndrome. The body usually has no problem and the brain can cope with one-two hours of sleep loss. However, traveling across 3 time zones or more is going to become a problem, and anyone who has traveled through more than six time zones always has a problem adapting to local time. This is because the brain is isolated and continues to follow the "usual" circadian rhythm. It is similar to being in a room with no clock on the wall and there is no sunlight. Surprisingly, left without the usual day-night cues (like sunlight, clocks, etc), the brain will experience a 25-hour day. It effectively stretches out the day to a 25 hr circadian cycle. This is why it is easier to travel west than it is to go east across time zones. When you travel west, you are gaining extra hours but when you are going east, you are losing hours. A good example is when you travel from California to New York, west coast to east coast, where you lose three hours and suddenly find you have a 21-hour day. The brain will be "delayed" in relation to the clock (and sunlight), so when everyone is waking up at 7AM, your brain will act like it is 4AM! This also gives the brain less time to adapt and do the things it normally does from its own internal clock because when it is 8 pm and the sun sets, the brain is "delayed" back at

4 pm. Where did the day go! Everyone is getting tired and I'm wide awake!

What can be done to reduce the effects of jet lag? When you travel across a lot of time zones the most important thing to do is make sure you get enough sleep. You don't want to start a trip sleep deprived or tired. So, make sure you get plenty of sleep for a few days before traveling. Second most important thing is preparation for the move into the new time zones to give yourself and your brain time to adapt. So, if you are going east which involves six time zones, you should start going to bed earlier at night and getting up earlier in the morning. The earlier you get up, the earlier you will go to bed but you have to do this slowly so that you are not deprived of sleep. The worst thing you can do is to try and change your sleep pattern the day before you travel. You should avoid drinking alcohol as that disrupts your sleep and you also have to avoid getting dehydrated, as air travel normally causes dehydration. You should also expose yourself to sunlight, especially morning light at your new destination. If you are traveling east, you can self-medicate by buying melatonin over the counter. Some studies have shown that taking 1 to 3 mg at bedtime can help you fall asleep & possibly help reset your circadian rhythm. Alternatively, you can ask your physician to prescribe a short course of sleeping pills to help you sleep because you will not be able to sleep until the middle of the night. These problems are transient and will only be temporary if you treat them. If you go with the flow and be patient, you will find that your brain will adapt to the new time zone. It will gradually do this without intervention when you are exposed to sunlight and darkness; if you are travelling through five time zones it takes about three days to adapt. Adapting to "jet lag" is more difficult as you get older, probably more noticeable after age 60.

ABZZZ's of Sleep

CHAPTER 8- PARASOMNIAS

Parasomnias are the unusual things that can happen to people when they are asleep. This is because although they are not abnormal, some of them are bizarre. These things include sleep walking, talking in your sleep, nightmares and sleep terrors, all of which are familiar to a lot of parents.

Another disorder that is not as common is known as REM behavior disorder. This is where people act out their dreams in their sleep. The main difference between REM behavior disorder (RBD) and the other Parasomnias is that RBD happens when a person is in a dream sleep, while the others occur during "deep" sleep. Sleep walking, talking in your sleep, nightmares and sleep terrors are all quite common, especially during childhood, and most people have heard of them or seen people with them. They are frequently featured in movies and on television, but REM behavior is less common and not many people have heard of it. Now, "deep" sleep is the best stage of sleep you can get as the body is the most relaxed and the brainwaves, heart rate and metabolism are at their slowest. It is the most restful a person can be, and it is also the hardest sleep to wake someone from.

People experience walking, talking and night terrors when they are in "deep" sleep. They look as if they are awake when in fact they are deeply asleep. Another telltale sign is that because, generally, you get your deep sleep during the first half of the night and the dream sleep during the second half, the non-REM parasomnias usually happen in the first half of the night. Both parasomnias and "deep" sleep are more common during childhood, with sleep walking being considered a "normal" developmental occurrence because of this relationship. When a child is growing they need a lot of deep sleep because it is during this stage of sleep that the brain squirts out the growth hormone that allows the child's muscles, bones and body to grow. The parasomnias like sleep walking and night terrors occur when children go quickly from awake into deep sleep (instead of the normal more gradual descent down through "light" sleep) such that their brains and bodies do not co-ordinate. The body remains awake but the brain has entered the slow brain waves of "deep" sleep and is "deeply" unconscious. The body muscles are still closer to being awake, and if you were to lift a child out of bed when he or she is in deep sleep and stand them up, they would automatically start walking like a robot as the legs follow the repetition of walking. Meanwhile, the child remains deeply asleep. This is what is called "automatic" behavior. The eyes would be wide open and they would appear awake and "responsible", but they actually would be no more awake than a wind-up toy. This is the main danger of these developmental parasomnias in children; the environment needs to be "child-proof" like that of a toddler as the sleep walker cannot protect himself from any danger, including objects in their path. A sleep walker can behave as if they are awake by walking and avoiding some objects, opening doors, and even going up and down stairs, all without waking up! However, they are not "responsible" for their actions. Criminal acts have even been committed during a sleep walking episode and the courts usually don't convict the sleeper.

Sleep talking is another example of a parasomnia during which the sleeper will talk or babble while in "deep" sleep. He or she may sound like they are in meaningful conversation, but they are not conscious and have no control over what they are saying. It usually only lasts for a few minutes. The fact that these parasomnias are more common during childhood is because of the higher demand for "deep" sleep in the growing child. The more frequent and problematic the occurrence in a child implies the need for an added pressure for "deep" sleep in them, such as when they are "overtired" or sleep deprived.

Sleep terrors are more dramatic and can be even quite frightening to the observer. A sleep terror is an occurrence during "deep" sleep whereby the "sleeper" suddenly sits upright and starts crying or screaming in a "frightened state". Their eyes are open, they are sweating and trembling, their hearts racing, their breathing rate is very fast, and there is "fear in their eyes". They are usually speaking incoherently about something and may appear to be visually hallucinating. Most importantly, they CANNOT be consoled. Verbal reassurance doesn't affect them and physical contact like hugging may actually instill more fear in them. For a parent or guardian, seeing a child having sleep terror is a very uncomfortable experience because you seem very helpless. It is very important to "be there' for the child and assure that they do not injure themselves. Gentle reassurance and limited physical contact may be of some benefit. It is a self- limited episode, but may reoccur soon after they fall back asleep. Fortunately, another telltale sign that this is a parasomnia is that sleepers WILL NOT remember the occurrence in the morning. There is never any memory created during "deep" sleep, regardless of the length of the episode.

Sleep walking and sleep terrors are most common from age 4 through 12, with reports of anywhere from 5 to 15 % in all children. It occurs most commonly during the 1st hour of sleep, but can occur or recur anytime during the first 3 to 4 hours of sleep. By far, the most common cause is relative sleep deprivation; frequently, this is seen during holidays or after "sleepovers" when children are allowed to stay up later than usual. Children usually out-grow this condition. Sleep walking and sleep talking can continue in 1% of adults. It can occur for the first time in an adult due to relative sleep deprivation caused by medication, acute illness, another underlying sleep disorder like sleep apnea, alcohol, sedatives, or mental illness. There can be a related anxiety or stress.

A parasomnia seen mostly in adults is "bruxism" or teeth grinding. This happens when a person grinds their teeth back and forth while they sleep; they are usually unaware of it, but it is very bothersome to the bed partner. It can lead to worn and fractured teeth, along with headaches and jaw pain. While it is usually accompanied by anxiety and stress, it does not mean that there is an underlying psychological disorder.

So what should parents do in this situation? The main thing is to try to ensure the child gets enough sleep by enforcing an earlier bedtime. Sometimes it is not due to lack of sleep but simply because the developing child needs more sleep than normal. Not all children are alike in their sleep needs. As always, a parent needs to "prepare" the child for going to bed an hour or so before the actual bedtime.

While nightmares constitute one of the many parasomnias considered to be normal and part of the development of a child. The "REM

Behavior Disorder" (RBD) happens when a sleeper physically "acts out" their dream. Typically, it occurs in an elderly person with an underlying heart or circulation problem where the blood supply to the brain is compromised. So, people suffering from an atherosclerosis or on those on medication that affects their blood pressure or blood flow can possibly act out their dreams. Men or women will sometimes beat, fight or even try to strangle their spouse in the night without them knowing it. When they wake up from sleep, they will say that they saw someone trying to hurt them and they were just trying to fight them off or that there was a monster in bed with them and they were trying to choke it. It is hard to believe their story but research into REM behavior in sleep laboratories has proved these stories to be true because the agitated sleeper will always be in REM or "dream" sleep when this occurs.

REM behavior disorder is a very scary problem because sufferers can hurt themselves or someone else as they experience it without realizing what they are doing. Luckily, the condition is treatable and doctors will try to better treat the underlying heart condition or the blood vessel problem. Alternatively, they will use a medication that limits the amount of dream sleep a person gets which can lessen the occurrence.

CHAPTER 9- INSOMNIA SYMPTOMS AND BASIC TREATMENT METHODS

The 3 types of Insomnia
1 **Sleep-onset Insomnia:** is usually associated with anxiety or "normal" daytime stress. There is usually an identifiable event which triggered the beginning of the patient's insomnia. A job change, relationship change, death or birth in the family, all are examples of situational stress which can initiate a difficulty in falling asleep as one "takes the situation to bed with them."
2 **Sleep maintenance Insomnia:** is a result of many different disorders. The sleeper can awaken during the normal course of sleep(remember we wake up every 60-90 minutes) but will have increased thoughts that prevent the resumption of sleep which should usually happen after several minutes. There is also more non-Primary insomnia causes in this category of Insomnia. This would include other sleep disorders like Sleep Apnea or Periodic Leg Movements of Sleep.
3 **Early morning awakening Insomnia:**is when a sleeper wakes up 2-3 hours earlier than the desired time and then lies there in bed without being able to fall back asleep. This is a classic symptom of depression.

3 broad Categories of Insomnia causes
1 **Primary Insomnia:** is insomnia without any other medical, psychiatric, or sleep disorder association.

2 **Co-morbid Medical Condition Insomnia:** is insomnia due to a medical condition like gastro-esophageal reflux which causes heartburn that awakens the sleep, or diabetes which causes frequent urination during the night.

3 **Co-morbid sleep disorder Insomnia:** is insomnia due to another sleep disorder like Sleep Apnea or Periodic Leg Movements of Sleep.

Treatment Methods

There are four components to any therapeutic approach to controlling insomnia. "Controlling" insomnia is probably a better term for the treatment of chronic insomnia compared to "curing", because chronic insomnia is usually a lifetime problem that is brought out by some stress in life. Therefore, it is usually likely to return and teaching a patient to be able to recognize and control the factors propagating their insomnia is more realistic than "finding a magic bullet" to instantly resolve it. Although the initial work-up of a person with insomnia will most likely look for any factor which may be easily resolved. These components are all equally important, as neglecting any one of them will only result in recurrence of sleepless nights. They are: **Sleep Hygiene; Sleep Restriction,Stimulus Control Therapy; Relaxation Therapy.**

Sleep Hygiene

Sleep Hygiene is something that everyone is better off knowing something about and probably consists of advice that you have heard before or seems rather common sense in origin. However, some sleep hygiene recommendations may actually debunk some old myths about what is good or bad for getting a good night's sleep. So this list of hygiene tips is both "negative" warnings and "positive" recommendations.

Sleep Hygiene Tips
• Do not drink coffee or caffeinated beverages without 5-6 hours of bedtime.
• Do not exercise within 3 hours of sleep. You may think that exercise may "tire you out", but actually exercise raises the body temperature and is a "stimulant" to the body. However, a short relaxing walk in the evening may be beneficial.
• Do not smoke cigarettes within 2 hours of bedtime. While the act of smoking may be relaxing, the nicotine in cigarettes is a stimulant and will make sleep more difficult.
• Do not "take your problems to bed." Don't wait until you are lying in bed to begin thinking about the consequences of your day or the demands of tomorrow.
• Do not do homework or work related problems in bed. Many people do this not only before going to bed, but as the last thing they do in bed before they turn the lights out. This stimulates the brain and doesn't allow for the necessary relaxation changes prior to falling asleep.
• Don't eat a large meal within 90 minutes of bedtime. However, eating a light snack is recommended to avoid hunger during the night.

- Keep a regular bedtime and wake time throughout the week.

- Exercise for at least 20 minutes in the morning or afternoon. Remember that exercise is anything that will use more muscular activity and raise your heart rate. Park farther away in the parking lot; use the stairs instead of the elevator.

- Get out in the open air and expose yourself to sunlight. This helps establish and strengthen the body's circadian rhythm or "inner clock."

- Do not drink alcohol with 3 hours of bedtime. (The VERY commonly used "night cap" is a bad choice if you are having trouble falling, and especially, staying asleep.).
- Don't expect any of these recommendations to instantly work or not help. However, following each of these recommendations for the long term on a regular basis is nearly "guaranteed" to improve your sleep.

Stimulus Control Therapy

This therapy is designed to stop the negative association between the bed and the undesirable outcomes such as wakefulness, worry and frustration. Usually, these negative feeling come about because of prolonged periods of wakefulness in bed during which there is added "effort" and pressure to fall asleep. Stimulus Control Therapy is intended to establish a clear line between the bed and sleep, thereby forming a regular sleep-wake cycle. Many of the important steps in Stimulus Control Therapy are included in sleep hygiene measures, but are more or less emphasized individually in therapy.

Sleep Control Measures	
1	Only go to bed when you are sleepy.
2	Do not nap during the day.
3	Do not lie in bed awake for more than 20 minutes at a time.
4	Do not use the bed for any work or studying.
5	Get up and out of bed promptly when you wake in the morning.

Self Restriction Therapy

Another way to accomplish a good night's sleep is to improve the "efficiency" of your time in bed. This is done by calculating or estimating the amount of time that you are sleeping every night. It is an amount that is (much) less than normal. Most people will spend 7-8 hours in bed, but will calculate that they are only sleeping for 4-6 hours. IN other words, they are awake in bed for 2-3 hours or more. With Sleep Restriction Therapy, a wake-up time is decided upon (usually depending on work, school, or family responsibilities) and the total sleep time is subtracted from this hour to determine the bedtime. For example, someone goes to bed at 10PM, gets up at 6 AM, but only sleeps 5 ½ hours each night. The SRT formula would start the new bedtime at 1:00 AM, which allows the same amount of sleep with an 85% efficiency, but would consolidate the sleep. This would further reinforce the bed with sleep as emphasized in Stimulus Control Therapy. Every5 to 7 days of adhering to the schedule, 15 minutes can be added to the bedtime until the desired amount of optimal time is achieved. Sleep restriction "almost always" works, but the difficult part is following the schedule on a regular basis and not going to bed too early.

Cognitive Behavioral Therapy

Cognitive Behavioral Therapy is a combination of cognitive (talking therapy), with behavioral treatment plans, like "Sleep Restriction" and Sleep Hygiene" methods. There may also be a need for ongoing "Relaxation Techniques", like hypnosis, sound machines, or "progressive muscle relaxation."The emphasis in Cognitive Therapy is to allow the patient to express his or her complaints, insights, concerns, or fears about their inability to sleep, and then to individually make corrections in their misperceptions. Examples are statements like, "If I can't sleep, I should just stay in bed and rest", or "I don't sleep at all", or "if I have a bad night's sleep, then I can't do anything the next day".

CONCLUSION

There are some things in life you cannot control. The people around you and other elements of the environment in which you live and work are among these things. How you respond to that environment is within your control, as is Insomnia.

Your approach to Insomnia should be a comprehensive one. You should not expect a simple, "take this pill or do this and you will sleep like a baby" approach. Facing and beating insomnia is best done as part of a "Living Healthier" lifestyle. You need to try to quantify how you are sleeping with a sleep diary for at least 2 weeks. This will give you a more realistic "score" of how you are sleeping. Then a commitment to improving your general health is needed. Adopt a good sleep hygiene, eat better, exercise on a regular basis, quit smoking, limit alcohol intake and over the counter medication. Speak to your physician about the use or abuse of prescribed sleep medication. Stay committed; stay true to your plan and yourself. Be optimistic, because there is a better way and a better night's sleep ahead.

RECOMMENDED READING

In over three decades of studying sleep —its purpose, mechanics and how to help those who are in need of it, I have gathered, read and researched upon lots of content that would help me enlighten and broaden my knowledge and understanding. Below are some of the materials that have enriched my learning further. I earnestly hope these books will do the same for you. You can check them out on my site here:

http://SleepDisordersInformation.org/recommended

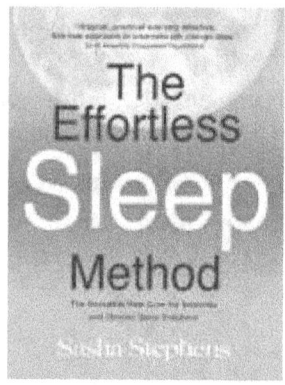

The Effortless Sleep Method: The Incredible New Cure for Insomnia and Chronic Sleep Problems

This book is what every insomniac needs. With very original, practical and effective sleep tips guaranteed to give you an effortless sleep.

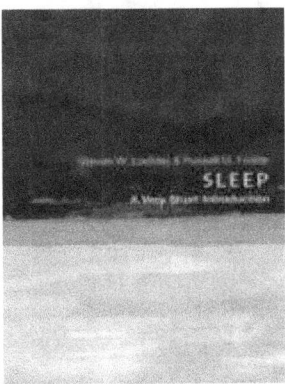

Sleep: A Very Short Introduction

We spend almost around a third of our lives asleep. When know that it's vital to our health and bodily functions. But just how much sleep is actually considered "healthy"? This book will provide answers to a whole lot of sleep related questions.

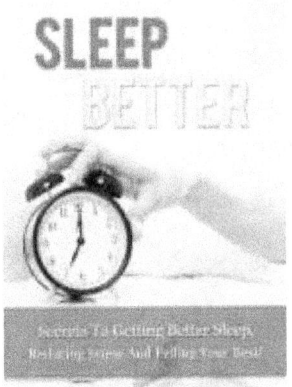

Sleep Better: Secrets To Getting Better Sleep, Reducing Stress, And Feeling Your Best! (Sleep Better, sleeping disorders)

Reach your goal towards getting better sleep quality with methodical strategies and tested steps. Reduce your stress and feel your best each and every single time you wake up.

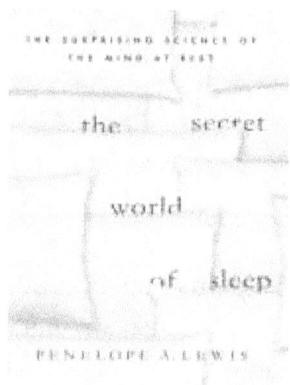

The Secret World of Sleep: The Surprising Science of the Mind at Rest (MacSci)

This book provides the latest research on sleep, resting and how to get more of both by laying simple truth and information. Authored by an authority in the field of sleep, Lewis fills in the gaps to uncovering and learning the secret world of sleep.

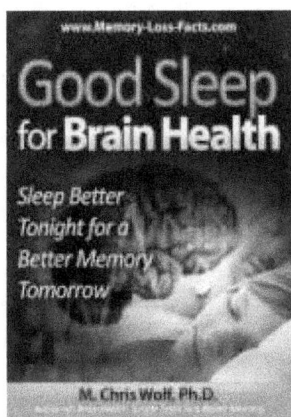

Good Sleep for Brain Health: Sleep Better Tonight for a Better Memory Tomorrow

A healthy brain for a better memory. Get a good night's sleep with the help of this book and improve your body's overall health and at the same time, boost your brain's capacity for memory retention.

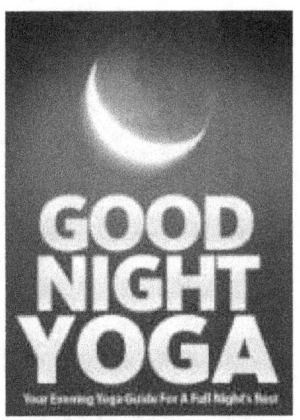

Good Night Yoga: Your Evening Yoga Guide For A Full Night's Rest (Just Do Yoga)

Sleep well to Good Night Yoga. Yes, you heard right! This book holds powerful Yoga relaxation routine and techniques to soothe and calm yourself in preparation for a good night's rest.

ABOUT THE AUTHOR

Dr Kohan was educated at the University Of Virginia where he also received his M.D. from the School of Medicine. He finished his residency training at Long Island College Hospital in Brooklyn, NYC.

Dr Kohan completed a fellowship in Pulmonary Medicine at the University of Rochester. He finished sleep medicine training at St. Mary's Sleep Center in Rochester, NY, which at the time was one of only five sleep labs in the U.S.

Dr. Kohan has founded and directed sleep labs throughout the world, including New Hartford, NY; Ljubljana, Slovenia; Honolulu and Hilo, HI: PagoPago,Am. Samoa; Anchorage, AK; San Diego and El Centro, CA. He has seen the field of sleep medicine grow from a medical curiosity to one of everyday recognition.

You can find Dr. Kohan on Google+ and Facebook.